The 36 Superfoods for Weight Loss

Get Started on Healthy Living by Eating Right

By: Billy Joseph

9781681279459

I0711643

PUBLISHERS NOTES

Disclaimer – Speedy Publishing LLC

This publication is intended to provide helpful and informative material. It is not intended to diagnose, treat, cure, or prevent any health problem or condition, nor is intended to replace the advice of a physician. No action should be taken solely on the contents of this book. Always consult your physician or qualified health-care professional on any matters regarding your health and before adopting any suggestions in this book or drawing inferences from it.

The author and publisher specifically disclaim all responsibility for any liability, loss or risk, personal or otherwise, which is incurred as a consequence, directly or indirectly, from the use or application of any contents of this book.

Any and all product names referenced within this book are the trademarks of their respective owners. None of these owners have sponsored, authorized, endorsed, or approved this book.

Always read all information provided by the manufacturers' product labels before using their products. The author and publisher are not responsible for claims made by manufacturers.

This book was originally printed before 2014. This is an adapted reprint by Speedy Publishing LLC with newly updated content designed to help readers with much more accurate and timely information and data.

Speedy Publishing LLC

40 E Main Street, Newark, Delaware, 19711

Contact Us: 1-888-248-4521

Website: http://www.speedypublishing.co

REPRINTED Paperback Edition: 9781681279459:

Manufactured in the United States of America

DEDICATION

This book is dedicated to my wonderful little girl, Sophia

Table of Contents

Chapter 1- Being Overweight is Not a Sin

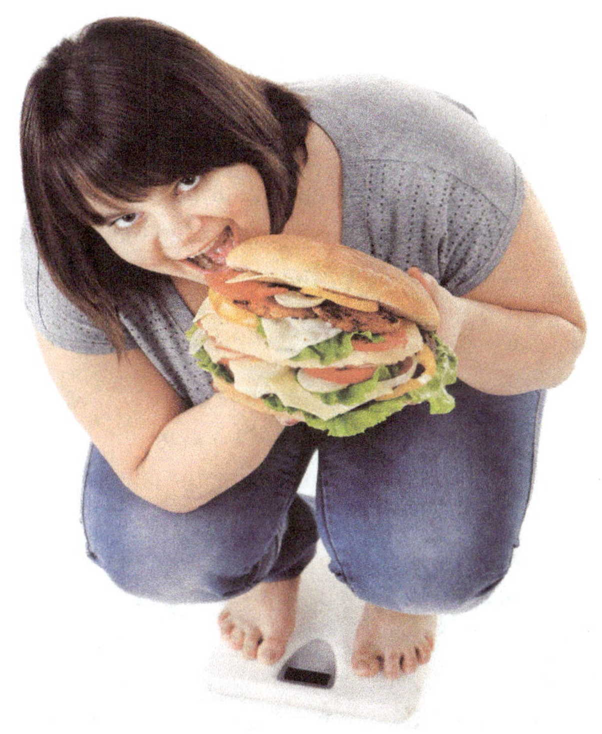

If you're overweight, you are not a bad person. You're simply overweight. But it's important to lose the extra pounds so you'll look good, feel healthier and develop a sense of pride and self-esteem. Once you've lost the fat, you'll need to maintain your weight. Most Americans pack on those extra pounds by eating the wrong things. Changing these poor eating habits is the key to long-term success. Knowledge – along with the right food – is the key.

When humans lived in caves, they didn't know anything about preserving and storing food. They spent all their waking time and energy hunting and gathering food. When they had it, they gobbled it down fast. Instead of storing food in pantries or cupboards, they stored energy in their bodies in the form of fat to burn during periods when there was little or nothing to eat. Each year, it was absolutely vital for them to put on a good layer of fat during the warm spring and summer months.

That was the only way they could guarantee their survival during the lean and mean winter months. And since women bore the young, they needed more energy to sustain themselves and their babies, and that meant they were usually heavier. Even though we no longer live in caves, we have inherited and maintained this basic mechanism for fat storage from our hunting and gathering ancestors.

Each one of us is born with a certain number of fat cells. How many of these fat cells you possess depend on genetics. If you have a lot of fat cells, maybe your ancestors were the biggest people in the tribe, which was a good thing because they had the best chances of survival. You can never get rid of fat cells, but – unfortunately – you can add to them.

Depending upon what you eat, your body will manufacture new far cells. And like those you were born with, they never go away. That doesn't mean you're doomed to be fat once you put on extra pounds. It is possible to shrink fat cells. That's what happens when you lose weight. You burn up the fat stored in those big fat cells.

Think of them as balloons. Burning off the fat inside them has the same effect as letting the air out of a balloon. A good weight loss program requires a certain amount of intake restriction – the consumption of fewer calories. You burn off the fat by eating less fat and becoming more active. To guarantee a lifetime of weight-control success, you have to change the type of foods you eat, so that you ingest less fat and still get the vitamins, minerals, trace elements, protein, fat and carbohydrates your body needs to thrive.

Extremely low-calorie diets may help you shed pounds quickly, but they'll lead to failure in the long run. That's because humans are genetically protected against starvation. During food shortages, our bodies slow down our metabolisms and burn less energy so we can stay alive.

A part of our brain called the hypothalamus keeps us on an even weight keep by creating a "set point." That's the weight where we feel comfortable. The hypothalamus determines this point based on the level of consumption it's used to. It seeks to keep our weight constant, even if that point is over what it should be. When we drastically cut back our food intake, the brain thinks the body is starving, and in an effort to preserve life, it slows the metabolism. Soon the pounds stop coming off.

Consequently, we grow hungry and uncomfortable and then eat more. And then the diet fails. How can you compensate for this metabolic slow-down? The answer is that you have to change the nutritional composition of the foods you eat. You will have to cut down on total calories – that's absolutely basic to weight loss.

More important, however, is reducing the percentage of total calories you are getting from fat. That's how you'll avoid starvation panic in your system. At the same time, you reduce the amount of fat in your food, replacing it with safe, low calorie, nutrient-rich plant foods. This will convince your brain that your body is getting all the nutrition it needs.

In fact, you'll be able to eat more food and feel more satisfied while consuming fewer calories and fats. Plant foods break down slowly in your stomach, making you feel full longer, and they are rich in vitamins, minerals, trace elements, carbohydrates and protein for energy and muscle-building. This allows your body to burn off its excess stored fat.

The Quick Fat Burners

Each one of the following foods is clinically proven to promote weight loss. These foods go a step beyond simply adding no fat to your system – they possess special properties that add zip to your system and help your body melt away unhealthy pounds. These incredible foods can suppress your appetite for junk food and keep your body running smoothly with clean fuel and efficient energy. You can include these foods in any sensible weight-loss plan. They give your body the extra metabolic kick that it needs to shave off weight quickly.

A sensible weight loss plan calls for no fewer than 1,200 calories per day. But Dr. Charles Klein recommends consuming more than that, if you can believe it – 1,500 to 1,800 calories per day. He says you will still lose weight quite effectively at that intake level without endangering your health. Hunger is satisfied more completely by filling the stomach. Ounce for ounce, the foods listed below accomplish that better than any others. At the same time, they're rich in nutrients and possess special fat-melting talents.

CHAPTER 2- THE NUTRITION FOUNDATION

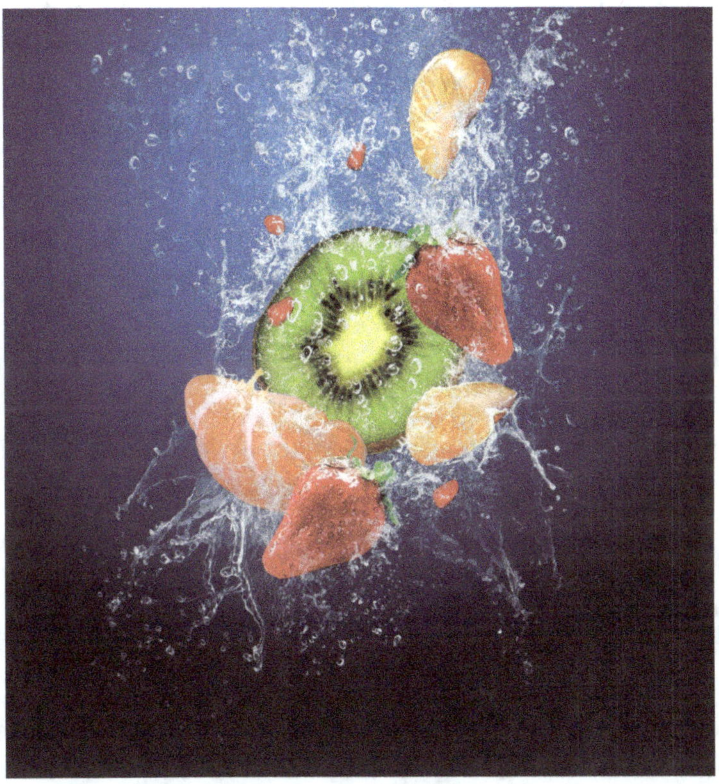

A healthy nutritional diet requires being well rounded with the suitable amount of nutrients, vitamins as well as minerals. The RDA's recommendation for day-to-day consumption of such things is a good place to check your optimal intakes.

The first thing that you should know about nutrition is this information: Consuming little meals every few hours will boost your metabolism and reduce fat storage. This is a proven fact that muscle-builders, models, athletes and thin people generally follow - you should give it a try as well.

Consuming the proper foods once you wake up is critical when breaking the fast your body goes into nightly. Approximately 3-4 hours after you eat your body shuts down your metabolism and behaves as though it is required to store food. This is a great function to possess if a shortage erupts and you do not see food for a long period of time. After all, if there is a shortage you're going to need your body to work "efficiently" by stashing away fat, and burning it as little as possible.

Nevertheless, you don't desire your body to stock up on fat and burn it slowly now, correct? Because there's no food shortage or famine at the time being (and more than likely won't be one in the near future) then it's pretty irritating when your body begins loading up on the pounds. So, in order to communicate with your body that it's fit, well-nourished, and not in demand of additional fat storage you need to reprogram your metabolism.

Here's the way you do it. Begin your day off with a little meal and continue to eat small meals every few hours throughout the day.

What should you eat? Here I'm simply going to give you general guidelines - because we would have to sit down together to make a precise fat burning diet plan for your body. These suggestions are a basic guideline to healthy types of food that don't boost fat storage.

• Protein: 35%

• Fat: 25%

• Carbs: 40%

All meals that you eat should contain calories coming from protein, carbs and fat. Your body is required to consume each of these in small portions throughout the day - as you take in a meal that's 90% carbohydrate 5% fat and 5% protein your body is going to digest it quicker (i.e. feel hungry again quicker) even if the calorie count is the same as a meal with above percentages, and you have more potential to stash away a percentage of the carbs as fat.

Hang on...

Do not go and get rid of the carbs out of your meals quite yet. Trimming down carbs could cause your body to once more enter fat storage mode. Trust me, you don't need that.

The Need to Eat Well

Why do I need to eat healthy food?

Regardless of when you begin, eating a healthy diet can assist you in maintaining and even improving your health - even more so if you combine it with exercise as well.

Putting together, healthy eating habits and routine physical activity can be the difference between independence and a life of being able to do nothing on your own.

This can aid you in life by providing you with the energy you require to remain active and do the things you wish to do. As well, healthy eating can also stop or slow down the advancement of numerous chronic sicknesses, such as heart disease and diabetes, osteoporosis and a few types of cancer. Eating healthy can also help you deal better with both physical and mental strain, operations and even the common cold or influenza.

The Link between Graceful Aging and Healthy Nutrition

Healthy living - which includes both consuming healthy food and maintaining a regular exercise routine - can assist you in conforming to the natural maturing process and keep your youthful vigor.

The Foundation of Healthy Living

Consume an assortment of foods. Eat in moderation. Size matters, so limit your portions!

Consume a lot of:

• Veggies and fruit

• Whole grains (for example, breads, pasta, oatmeal and brown rice)

• Legumes (such as dried beans, peas, lentils)

• Sea Food

• Unsaturated fats (from vegetable oils, nuts, and seeds)

• Lean meat (for example chicken and turkey)

• Consume Less:

• Saturated fats (found in butter, lard, deli meats, bacon and

• sausages)

• Trans fats (found in processed foods, cookies, cakes and deep-fried foods)

- Refined or enriched grains

- Salt and sugar (including sugary drinks as well as jams, candies

- and baked goods)

- Consume a lot of water.

- Participate in something active daily.

Go Against the Popular Eating Fashion

The difficult part is to eat in a fashion that aids you in maintaining a healthy weight, while also providing you with the nutrients you require for good health.

- Veggies and fruit

- Grain products, including bread rice, pasta and cereals

- Milk and alternatives like low fat cheese and yogurt

- Meat - fish, shellfish, poultry, lean meat - and alternatives, like eggs, beans, lentil, chickpeas, tofu and nuts.

Reality-Focused Goals

The simplest method to move towards consuming healthy food daily is to set goals that you truly can meet. For instance, say to yourself:

- I'll eat one more fruit and one more veggie today.

- I'll try a fruit or vegetable this week that I have never tried before.

- I'll eat fish once this week.

- I'll choose whole grain bread for my sandwich.

- I'll drink one more glass of water each day.

- I'll be more active today.

- I'll throw out my deep fryer.

- I'll do most of my shopping around the outer edges of the grocery store, because that's where the fresh foods are.

A couple of small changes can rise up to a very big difference to your health - before you even know it's happening!

CHAPTER 3- WHAT FOODS BURN FATS FAST?

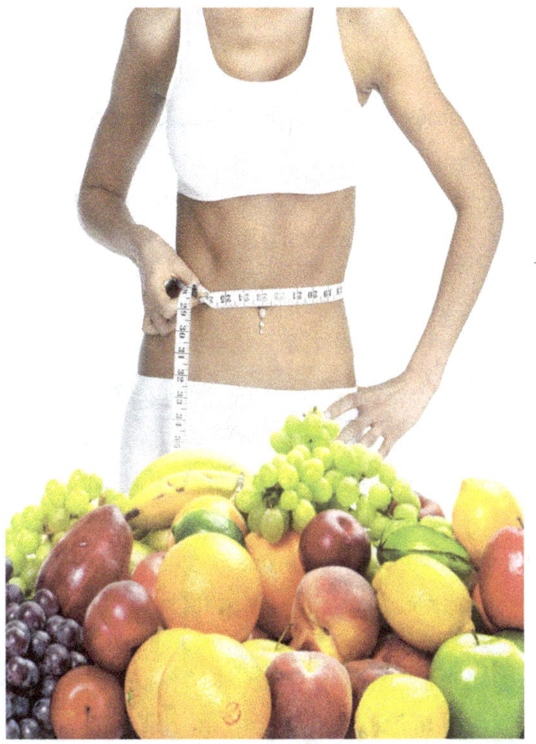

• **Fruits**

Apples

These marvels of nature deserve their reputation for keeping the doctor away when you eat one a day. And now, it seems, they can help you melt the fat away, too.

First of all, they elevate your blood glucose (sugar) levels in a safe, gentle manner and keep them up longer than most foods. The practical effect of this is to leave you feeling satisfied longer, say researchers.

Secondly, they're one of the richest sources of soluble fiber in the supermarket. This type of fiber prevents hunger pangs by guarding against dangerous swings or drops in your blood sugar level, says Dr. James Anderson of the University of Kentucky's School of Medicine.

An average size apple provides only 81 calories and has no sodium, saturated fat or cholesterol. You'll also get the added health benefits of lowering the level of cholesterol already in your blood as well as lowering your blood pressure.

Grapefruit

There's good reason for this traditional diet food to be a regular part of your diet. It helps dissolve fat and cholesterol, according to Dr. James Cerd of the University of Florida. An average sized grapefruit has 74 calories, delivers a whopping 15 grams of pectin (the special fiber linked to lowering cholesterol and fat), is high in vitamin C and potassium and is free of fat and sodium.

It's rich in natural galacturonic acid, which adds to its potency as a fat and cholesterol fighter. The additional benefit here is assistance in the battle against atherosclerosis (hardening of the arteries) and the development of heart disease. Try sprinkling it with cinnamon rather than sugar to take away some of the tart taste.

• Vegetables and Spices

Peppers

Hot, spicy chili peppers fall into the same category as hot mustard, Henry says. He studied them under the same circumstances as the mustard and they worked just as well. A mere three grams of chili peppers were added to a meal consisting of 766 total calories. The peppers' metabolism-raising properties worked like a charm, leading to what Henry call a diet-induced thermic effect. It doesn't take much to create the effect. Most salsa recipes call for four to eight chilies – that's not a lot.

Peppers are astonishingly rich in vitamins A and C, abundant in calcium, phosphorus, iron and magnesium, high in fiber, free of fat, low in sodium and have just 24 calories per cup.

Potatoes

We've got to be kidding, right? Wrong. Potatoes have developed the same "fattening" rap as bread, and it's unfair. Dr. John McDougal, director of the nutritional medicine clinic at St. Helena Hospital in Deer Park, California, says, "An excellent food with which to achieve rapid weight loss is the potato, at 0.6 calories per gram or about 85 calories per potato." A great source of fiber and potassium, they lower cholesterol and protect against strokes and heart disease.

Preparation and toppings are crucial. Steer clear of butter, milk and sour cream, or you'll blow it. Opt for yogurt instead.

Spinach

Popeye really knew what he was talking about, according to Dr. Richard Shekelle, an epidemiologist at the University of Texas. Spinach has the ability to lower cholesterol, rev up the metabolism and burn away fat. Rich in iron, beta carotene and vitamins C and E, it supplies most of the nutrients you need.

Whole Grain Bread

You needn't dread bread. It's the butter, margarine or cream cheese you put on it that's fattening, not the bread itself. We'll say this as often as needed – fat is fattening. If you don't believe that, ponder this – a gram of carbohydrate has four calories, a gram of protein four, and a gram of fat nine. So which of these is really fattening?

Bread, a natural source of fiber and complex carbohydrates, is okay for dieting. Norwegian scientist Dr. Bjarne Jacobsen found that people who eat less than two slices of bread daily weigh about 11 pounds more that those who eat a lot of bread.

Studies at Michigan State University show some bread actually reduce the appetite. Researchers compared white bread to dark, high-fiber bread and found that students who ate 12 slices a day of the dark, high-fiber bread felt less hunger on a daily basis and lost five pounds in two months. Others who ate white bread were hungrier, ate more fattening foods and lost no weight during this time.

So the key is eating dark, rich, high-fiber breads such as pumpernickel, whole wheat, mixed grain, oatmeal and others. The average slice of whole grain bread contains only 60 to 70 calories, is rich in complex carbohydrates – the best, steadiest fuel you can give your body – and delivers surprising amount of protein.

Coffee

Easy does it is the password here. We've all heard about potential dangers of caffeine – including anxiety and insomnia – so moderation is the key.

The caffeine in coffee can speed up the metabolism. In nutritional circles, it's known as a metabolic enhancer, according to Dr. Judith Stern of the University of California at Davis.

This makes sense, since caffeine is a stimulant. Studies show it can help you burn more calories than normal, perhaps up to 10 percent more. For safety's sake, it's best to limit your intake to a single cup in the morning and one in the afternoon. Add only skim milk to tit and try doing without sugar – many people learn to love it that way.

Mustard

Try the hot, spicy kind you find in Asian import stores, specialty shops and exotic groceries. Dr. Jaya Henry of Oxford Polytechnic Institute in England, found that the amount of hot mustard normally called for in Mexican, Indian and Asian recipes, about one teaspoon, temporarily speeds up the metabolism, just as caffeine and the drug ephedrine do.

"But mustard is natural and totally safe," Henry says. "It can be used every day, and it really works. I was shocked to discover it can speed up the metabolism by as much as 20 to 25 percent for several hours." This can result in the body burning an extra 45 calories for every 700 consumed, Dr. Henry says.

Rice

An entire weight-loss plan, simple called the Rice Diet, was developed by Dr. William Kempner at Duke University in Durham, North Carolina. The diet, dating to the 1930's, makes rice the staple of your food intake. Later on, you gradually mix in various fruits and vegetables.

It produces stunning weight loss and medical results. The diet has been shown to reverse and cure kidney ailments and high blood pressure.

A cup of cooked rice (150 grams) contains about 178 calories – approximately one-third the number of calories found in an equivalent amount of beef or cheese. And remember, whole grain rice is much better for you than white rice.

Soups

Soup is good for you! Maybe not the canned varieties from the store – but old-fashioned, homemade soup promotes weight loss. A study by Dr. John Foreyt of Baylor College of Medicine in Houston, Texas, found that dieters who ate a bowl of soup before lunch and dinner lost more weight than dieters who didn't. In fact, the more soup they ate, the more weight they lost. And soup eaters tend to keep the weight off longer.

Naturally, the type of soup you eat makes a difference. Cream soups or those made of beef or pork are not your best bets. But here's a great recipe:

Slice three large onions, three carrots, four stalks of celery, one zucchini and one yellow squash. Place in a kettle. Add three cans crushed tomatoes, two packets low-sodium chicken bouillon, three cans water and one cup white wine (optional). Add tarragon, basil, oregano, and thyme and garlic powder. Boil, and then simmer for an hour. Serves six.

Tofu

You just can't say enough about this health food from Asia. Also called soybean curd, it's basically tasteless, so any spice or flavoring you add blends with it nicely. A 2½" square has 86 calories and nine grams of protein. (Experts suggest an intake of about 40 grams per day.) Tofu contains calcium and iron, almost no sodium and not a bit of saturated fat. It makes your metabolism run on high and even lowers cholesterol. With different varieties available, the firmer tofu are goof for stir-frying or adding to soups and sauces while the softer ones are good for mashing, chopping and adding to salads.

Chapter 4- Fat-Fighting Foods that Work While You Eat

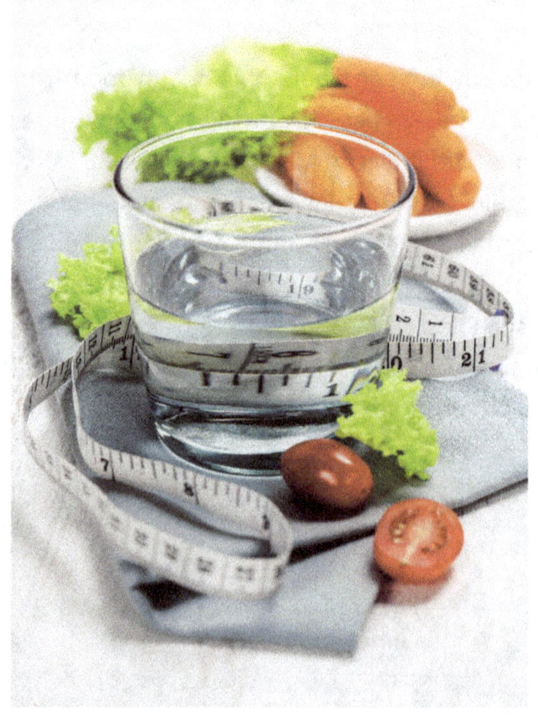

It would be unrealistic to think you could successfully lose weight and enjoy what you're eating with a mere handful of foods, no matter how delicious, nutritious and satisfying they may be. So we're going to add an extra roster of fat-fighting foods you can eat along with the great foods mentioned in the last section.

They'll lend different tastes and textures to every meal and provide a wide range of vitamins, minerals, proteins and other vital nutrients. Naturally, each one is high in fiber, low in fat and safe when it comes to sodium content, too.

Many have crunchiness and flavor we've come to desire in snack and nibbling foods. If you're like most of us, you may have a real junk food snacking habit – a habit you're going to have to change in order to slim down. Many of the foods in this section may be worthy substitutes.

• **Fruits**

Berries

This is the perfect weight-loss food. Berries have natural fructose sugar that satisfies your longing for sweets and enough fiber so you absorb fewer calories that you eat. British researchers found that the high content of insoluble fiber in fruits, vegetables and whole grains reduces the absorption of calories from foods enough to promote width loss without hampering nutrition.

Berries are a great source of potassium that can assist you in blood pressure control. Blackberries have 74 calories per cup, blueberries 81, raspberries 60 and strawberries 45. So use your imagination and enjoy the berry of your choice.

Figs

Fiber-rich figs are low in calories at 37 per medium (2.25" diameter) raw fig and 48 per dried fig. A recent study by the USDA demonstrated that they contribute to a feeling of fullness and prevent overeating. Subjects actually complained of being asked to eat too much food when fed a diet containing more figs than a similar diet with an identical number of calories.

Serve them with other fruits and cheeses. Or poach them in fruit juice and serve them warm or cold. You can stuff them with mild white cheese or puree them to use as a filling for cookies and low-calorie pastries.

The 36 Superfoods for Weight Loss
Kiwis

This New Zealand native is a sweet treat at only 46 calories per fruit. Chinese public health officials praise the tasty fruit for its high vitamin C content and potassium. It stores easily in the refrigerator for up to a month. Most people like it peeled, but the fuzzy skin is also edible.

Melons

Now, here's great taste and great nutrition in a low-calorie package! One cup of cantaloupe balls has 62 calories, on cup of casaba balls has 44 calories, one cup of honeydew balls has 62 calories and one cup of watermelon balls has 49 calories. They have some of the highest fiber content of any food and are delicious. Throw in handsome quantities of vitamins A and C plus a whopping 547 mgs of potassium in that cup of cantaloupe, and you have a fat-burning health food beyond compare.

Tomatoes

A medium tomato (2.5" diameter) has only about 25 calories. These garden delights are low in fat and sodium, high in potassium and rich in fiber.

A survey at Harvard Medical School found that the chances of dying of cancer are lowest among people who eat tomatoes (or strawberries) every week.

And don't overlook canned crushed, peeled, whole or stewed tomatoes. They make sauces, casseroles and soups taste great while retaining their nutritional goodness and low-calorie status. Even plain old spaghetti sauce is a fat-burning bargain when served over pasta, so think about introducing tomatoes into your diet.

• Vegetables

Broccoli

Broccoli is America's favorite vegetable, according to a recent poll. No wonder. A cup of cooked broccoli has a mere 44 calories. It delivers a staggering nutritional payload and is considered the number one cancer-fighting vegetable. It has no fat, loads of fiber, cancer fighting chemicals called indoles, carotene, 21 times the RDA of vitamin C and calcium.

Pay attention to the color when you're buying broccoli. The tiny florets should be rich green and free of yellowing. Stems should be firm.

Beans

Beans are one of the best sources of plant protein. Peas, beans and chickpeas are collectively known as legumes. Most common beans have 215 calories per cooked cup (lima beans go up to 260). They have the most protein with the least fat of any food, and they're high in potassium but low in sodium.

Plant protein is incomplete, which means that you need to add something to make it complete. Combine beans with a whole grain – rice, barley, wheat, corn – to provide the amino acids necessary to form a complete protein. Then you get the same top-quality protein as in meat with just a fraction of the fat.

Studies at the University of Kentucky and in the Netherlands show that eating beans regularly can lower cholesterol levels.

The most common complaint about beans is that they cause gas. Here's how to contain that problem, according to the U.S.

Department of Agriculture (USDA): Before cooking, rinse the beans and remove foreign particles, put in a kettle and cover with boiling water, soak for four hours or longer, remove any beans that float to the top, and then cook the beans in fresh water.

Cabbage

This Eastern Europe staple is a true wonder food. There are only 33 calories in a cup of cooked shredded cabbage, and it retains all its nutritional goodness no matter how long you cook it. Eating cabbage raw (18 calories per shredded cup), cooked, as sauerkraut (27 calories per drained cup) or coleslaw (calories depend on dressing) only once a week is enough to protect against colon cancer. And it may be a longevity-enhancing food. Surveys in the United States, Greece and Japan show that people who eat a lot of it have the least colon cancer and the lowest death rates overall.

Carrots

What list of health-promoting, fat-fighting foods would be complete without Bugs Bunny's favorite? A medium-sized carrot carries about 55 calories and is a nutritional powerhouse. The orange color comes from beta carotene, a powerful cancer-preventing nutrient (provitamin A).

Chop and toss them with pasta, grate them into rice or add them to a stir-fry. Combine them with parsnips, oranges, raisins, lemon juice, chicken, potatoes, broccoli or lamb to create flavorful dishes. Spice them with tarragon, dill, cinnamon or nutmeg. Add finely chopped carrots to soups and spaghetti sauce – they impart a natural sweetness without adding sugar.

Billy Joseph
Greens

We're talking collard, chicory, beet, kale, mustard, Swiss chard and turnip greens. They all belong to the same family as spinach, and that's one of the super-stars. No matter how hard you try, you can't load a cup of plain cooked greens with any more than 50 calories.

They're full of fiber, loaded with vitamins A and C, and free of fat. You can use them in salads, soups, casseroles or any dish where you would normally use spinach.

Leeks

These members of the onion family look like giant scallions, and are every bit as healthful and flavorful as their better-known cousins. They come as close to calorie-free as it gets at a mere 32 calories per cooked cup.

You can poach or broil halved leeks and then marinate them in vinaigrette or season with Romano cheese, fine mustard or herbs. They also make a good soup.

Lettuce

People think lettuce is nutritionally worthless, but nothing could be farther from the truth. You can't leave it out of your weight-loss plans, not at 10 calories per cup of raw romaine. It provides a lot of filling bulk for so few calories. And it's full of vitamin C, too. Go beyond iceberg lettuce with Boston, bibb and cos varieties or try watercress, arugula, radicchio, dandelion greens, purslane and even parsley to liven up your salads.

Onions

Flavorful, aromatic, inexpensive and low in calories, onions deserve a regular place in your diet. One cup of chopped raw onions has only 60 calories, and one raw medium onion (2.15" diameter) has just 42.

They control cholesterol, thin the blood, protect against cholesterol and may have some value in counteracting allergic reactions. Most of all, onions taste good and they're good for you.

Partially boil, peel and bake, basting with olive oil and lemon juice. You can also sauté them in white wine and basil, then spread over pizza. Or roast them in sherry and serve over paste.

Sweet Potatoes

You can make a meal out of them and not worry about gaining a pound – and you sure won't walk away from the table feeling hungry. Each sweet potato has about 103 calories. Their creamy orange flesh is one of the best sources of vitamin A you can consume.

You can bake steam or microwave them. Or add them to casseroles, soups and many other dishes. You can also flavor with lemon juice or vegetable broth instead of butter.

• **Grain**

Buckwheat

It's great for pancakes, breads, cereal, and soups or alone as a grain dish commonly called kasha. It has 155 calories per cooked cup. Research at the All India Institute of Medical Sciences shows diets including buckwheat lead to excellent blood sugar regulation, resistance to diabetes and lowered cholesterol levels. You cook buckwheat the same way you would rice or barley. Bring two to three cups of water to a boil, add the grain, cover the pan, turn down the heat and simmer for 20 minutes or until the water is absorbed.

Barley

This filling grain stacks up favorably to rice and potatoes. It has 170 calories per cooked cup, respectable levels of protein and fiber and relatively low fat. Roman gladiators ate this grain regularly for strength and actually complained when they had to eat meat.

Studies at the University of Wisconsin show that barley lowers cholesterol by up to 15 percent. It was also found that it has powerful anti-cancer agents. Israeli scientists say it cures constipation better than laxatives - and that can promote weight loss, too.

Use it as a substitute for rice in salads, pilaf or stuffing, or add to soups and stews. You can also mix it with rice for an interesting texture. Ground into flour, it makes excellent breads and muffins.

Corn

It's really a grain – not a vegetable – and is another food that's gotten a bum rap. People think it has little to offer nutritionally and that just isn't so. There are 178 calories in a cup of cooked kernels. It contains good amounts of iron, zinc and potassium, and University of Nebraska researchers say it delivers a high-quality of protein, too.

The 36 Superfoods for Weight Loss

The Tarahumara Indians of Mexico eat corn, beans and hardly anything else. Virgil Brown, M.D., of Mount Sinai School of Medicine in New York, points out that high blood cholesterol and cardiovascular heart disease are almost nonexistent among them.

Oats

A cup of oatmeal or oat bran has only 110 calories. And oats help you lose weight. Subjects in Dr. James Anderson's landmark 12-year study at the University of Kentucky lost three pounds in two months simply by adding 100 grams (3.5 ounces) of oat bran to their daily food intake and nothing else. Just don't expect oats alone to perform miracles – you have to eat a balanced diet for total health.

• Meat

Chicken

White meat contains 245 calories per four ounce serving and dark meat, 285. It's an excellent source of protein, iron, niacin and zinc. Skinned chicken is healthiest, but most experts recommend waiting until after cooking to remove it because the skin keeps the meat moist during cooking.

Fish

The health benefits of fish are greater than experts imagined – and they've always considered it a health food.

The calorie count in the average four-ounce serving of a deep-sea fish runs from a low of 90 calories in abalone to a high of 236 in herring. Water-packed tuna, for example, has 154 calories. It's hard to gain weight eating seafood.

As far back as 1985, articles in the New England Journal of Medicine showed a clear link between eating fish regularly and lower rates of heart disease. The reason is that oils in fish thin the blood, reduce blood pressure and lower cholesterol.

Dr. Joel Kremer, at Albany Medical College in New York, discovered that daily supplements of fish oil brought dramatic relief to the inflammation and stiff joints of rheumatoid arthritis.

Turkey

Give thanks to those pilgrims for starting the wonderful tradition of Thanksgiving turkey. It just so happens that this health food disguised as meat is good year-round for weight control.

A four-ounce serving of roasted white meat turkey has 177 calories and dark meat has 211.

Sadly, many folks are still unaware of the versatility and flavor of ground turkey. Anything hamburger can do, ground turkey can do at least as well, from conventional burgers to spaghetti sauce to meat loaf.

Some ground turkey contains skin which slightly increases the fat content. If you want to keep it really lean, opt for ground breast meat. But since this has no added fat, you'll need to add filler to make burgers or meat loaf hold together.

Four ounces of ground turkey has approximately 170 calories and nine grams of fat – about what you'd find in 2.5 teaspoons of butter or margarine. Incredibly, the same amount of regular ground beef (21% fat) has 298 calories and 23 grams of fat.

Buying turkey has become easy. It's no longer necessary to buy a whole bird unless you want to. Ground turkey is available fresh or frozen, as are individual parts of the bird, including drumsticks, thighs, breasts and cutlets.

• Dairy

Cottage Cheese

As long as we're talking about losing weight and fat-fighting foods, we had to mention cottage cheese.

Low-fat (2%) cottage cheese has 205 calories per cup and is admirably low in fat, while providing respectable amounts of calcium and the B vitamin riboflavin. Add spices such a dill, or garden fresh vegetable like scallions and chives for extra zip.

To make it sweeter, add raisins or one of the fruit spreads with no sugar added. You can also use cottage cheese in cooking, baking, fillings and dips where you would otherwise use sour cream or cream cheese.

Yogurt

The non-fat variety of plain yogurt has 120 calories per cup and low-fat, 144. It delivers a lot of protein and, like any dairy food, is rich in calcium and contains zinc and riboflavin.

Yogurt is handy as a breakfast food – cut a banana into it and add the cereal of your choice.

You can find ways to use it in other types of cooking, to – sauces, soups, dips, toppings, stuffing and spreads. Many kitchen gadget departments even sell a simple funnel for making yogurt cheese.

Yogurt can replace heavy creams and whole milk in a wide range of dishes, saving scads of fat and calories.

You can substitute half or all of the higher fat ingredients. Be creative. For example, combine yogurt, garlic powder, lemon juice, and a dash of pepper and Worcestershire sauce and use it to top a baked potato instead of piling on fat-laden sour cream.

Supermarkets and health food stores sell a variety of yogurts, many with added fruit and sugar. To control calories and fat content, buy plain non-fat yogurt and add fruit yourself. Apple butter or fruit spreads with little or no added sugar are an excellent way to turn plain yogurt into a delectable sweet treat.

- **Pasta**

The Italians had it right all along. A cup of cooked paste (without a heavy sauce) has only 155 calories and fits the description of a perfect starch-centered staple. Analysis at the American Institute of Baking shows pasta is rich in six minerals, including manganese, iron, phosphorus, copper, magnesium and zinc. Also be sure to consider whole wheat pastas, which are even healthier.

Chapter 5- A Balanced Meal is a Healthy Meal

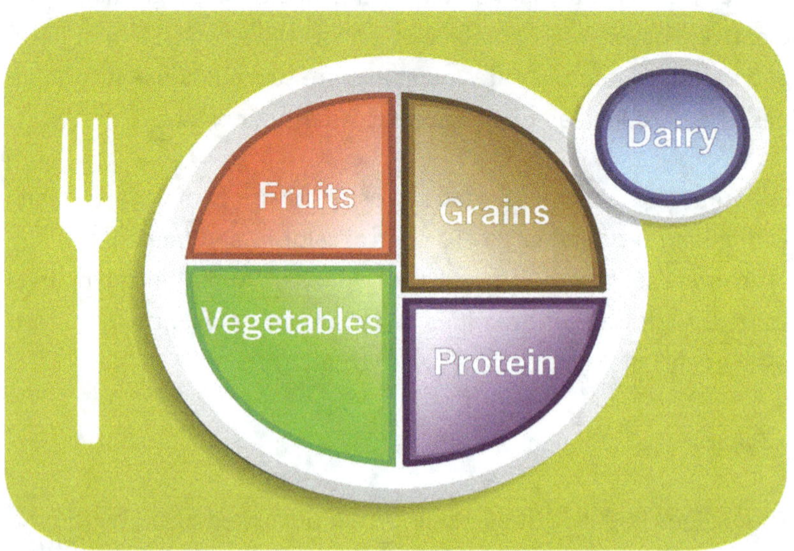

A nutrient is a substance that supplies nourishment necessary for life and growth. Eating healthy food is a significant method to make certain you acquire all the nutrients you need, with no additional calories or additional weight gain. If what you're eating doesn't provide you with adequate nutrition, you are able to take a multivitamin/mineral and/or other supplements to assist

Defining Healthy Eating

Healthy eating is balanced eating, where you eat an assortment of foods. It includes protein, carbs (especially fiber), fats and fluids.

Protein

Protein helps restore your muscular tissue, skin and nails. It can assist you in healing yourself if you have been sick or have had an operation. The greatest sources of protein include meat, fish, poultry, milk, eggs, cheese, yogurt, legumes (dried peas, beans and lentils for instance), nuts, seeds and soy products (tofu or soy beverages for instance).Whole grains, veggies and fruit can also supply little amounts of protein.

Here's how you are able to simply acquire the protein your body requires daily along with a lot of other good nutrients, like iron, calcium and vitamin B12:

- In the morning, consume a few egg whites as well as a piece of whole wheat toast and a banana. You can also try some oatmeal made with a few egg whites and milk or unsweetened, fortified soy beverage, or dry cereal make with low-fat buttermilk.

- In the afternoon, eat a piece of low fat cheese and some lentil soup. You might also want to try steamed brown rice with cut-up chicken chunks and veggies like green beans or bok choy.

- When snack time comes around, consume a handful of nuts with three-quarters of a cup of low-fat yogurt, or a little cup of milk or unsweetened, fortified soy beverage.

- At supper time, eat sea food (or tofu) with half a cup of brown or basmati rice, and half a cup of broccoli or other veggies and one cup of assorted salad.

Attempt to have a good source of protein at every meal. Try:

- Adding a piece of low fat cheese to your preferred sandwich

- Chopping up a hard-boiled egg and putting it into your salad

- Consuming a handful of unsalted soy nuts

- Scattering nuts and seeds on your cereal, salad or stir fry

- Scattering natural almond butter on a piece of whole wheat toast or a whole wheat tortilla

- Placing chickpeas or beans into a stir fry or pasta sauce.

- If you're still having difficulty acquiring sufficient protein through your eating habits, take a protein shake daily.

Carbs

Healthy carbs - like veggies, fruit, whole grains and low-fat dairy products - supply your body with the fuel your heart, lungs and additional organs need to operate properly. They have essential vitamins and minerals and assist you by giving you the energy you require to run another lap, swim a bit longer or to do an additional set of weight-lifts. Several are also crucial sources of fiber. A couple of carbs, nevertheless, are unhealthy- especially the ones that are easy to digest and that rapidly raise your blood sugar. These include white bread, white rice, cookies and cakes.

A few weight loss plans tell you to cut back on or get rid of all carbs since they make you put on more weight. Only that seriously restricts what you are able to consume and you lose out on numerous crucial nutrients.

Fiber

The majority of adults get only about 50% of the fiber they should be consuming every day. Fiber is a nutrient obtained from plants. In order to keep your bowels regular and healthy you are required to consume fiber. Consuming several high-fiber foods can also assist you to lower your blood cholesterol levels, maintain blood sugar levels and aid in preventing high blood pressure. Since fiber curves your appetite for longer periods of time, it can aid with weight control as well.

Grains and grain products are especially high in fiber levels. In reality, a high-fiber cereal for breakfast (one with four grams or more of fiber) will assist you in keeping your hunger in check for the entire day. Follow up throughout the day with additional high-fiber foods, like whole wheat toast or pasta with vegetable sauce, a hot bowl of chili, or low-fat yogurt with fruit and bran sprinkled on top. Fruits and veggies, beans, lentils and chickpeas are also excellent sources or fiber.

Fats

Studies now show that it's not fat that's unhealthy for you, but rather the kind of fat you consume that matters most. Everybody requires some fat to remain healthy. Fat supplies your body with vitality and aids in constructing a protective coat around your cells - but it must be healthy fat and in the correct portions.

Fats to avoid are saturated and Trans fats. Saturated fats are generally discovered in food that came from animals. Trans fats come generally from vegetable oils that have been made solid by a method named hydrogenation.

Unhealthy fats are found in:

- Whole or full - fat milk

- Cream, sour cream as well as ice cream

- Butter as well as clarified butter

- Cheese

• Fatty red meat (sausage, pork bacon, Chinese preserved meats)

• Chicken, duck as well as turkey skin of fat

• Hard margarines as well as vegetable shortening

• Partially hydrogenated vegetable oil

• Deep-fried foods

• Baked items (including cookies, cakes, pies and pastries)

Healthy fat are found in:

• Oily or fatty fish, such as salmon, anchovies, rainbow trout, sardines, mackerel, char and herring

• Nuts and seeds, such as cashews, almonds, walnuts, peanuts, and ground flaxseeds

• Vegetable oils, including olive, peanut, canola, soybean, and sesame oil

• Flaxseed as well as walnut oils (do not heat these oils; utilize them cold)

• Wheat germ

• Avocadoes

Foods strengthened with omega 3, including eggs, yogurt as well as soy beverage.

To make certain you're consuming the correct portion of fat, begin by picking foods that are naturally low in fat, and then add no more than two to three tablespoons (30 to 45 grams) of healthy, unsaturated fats to what you eat daily. This includes oil utilized for making food, salad dressings, margarine and mayonnaise.

As well, try to replace healthy fat for unhealthy fat wherever you are able to, and remember to study food labels cautiously. Low fat means that the food has less than three grams of fat per serving. Fat free means that the food has less than 0.5 grams of fat per serving.

Additionally:

• Choose lean meats, and then trim off all fat you are able to see.

• Take off the skin from chicken as well as turkey.

• Grill, broil or roast your meat, chicken or turkey to allow the fat to drain off.

• Eat fish two or more times a week.

• Choose legumes instead of meat at least once a week. Cook a dish that utilizes baked beans, lentils or chickpeas, or prepare a batch of chili.

• Cook with low-fat dairy products made with skim or 1% milk of yogurt.

• Utilize low-fat milk in your coffee and tea.

• Utilize some mustard, ketchup, relish, cranberry sauce, or natural almond butter instead of butter or margarine.

• Choose a healthy, low-fat salad dressing or create your own.

CHAPTER 6 – CAREFUL WITH THE SEASONING!

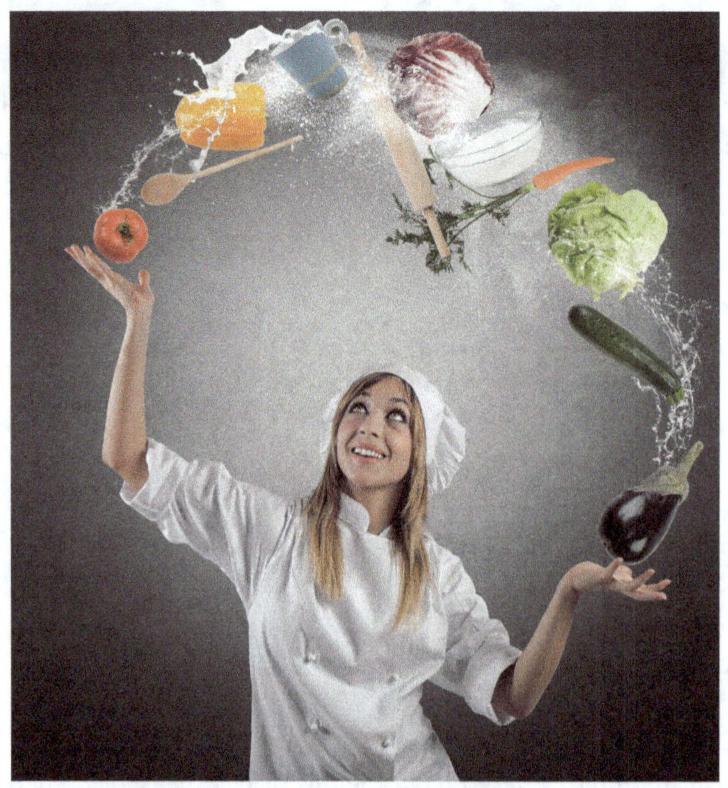

The brightest and most colorful vegetables and fruits - the dark green, orange, yellow and red ones - are jammed with both necessary vitamins and minerals and disease-fighting phytochemicals. Soy products, beans and lentils, as well, are full of phytochemicals - so remember to include them. And do not be concerned about seasoning your foods with herbs, spices and citrus peels to get additional nutrients.

What Does Salt Do?

You more than likely know that consuming an excessive amount of sodium (salt) may increase blood pressure, which may lead to heart disease. Only recent research exposes that the effects of high blood pressure are even more varied.

Investigators now recognize that high blood pressure may also accelerate the body's loss of calcium, which could lead to osteoporosis (thinning of the bones that cause them to break easily).High blood pressure is also believed to be a "risk factor" for diabetes and kidney disease, which implies you're more probable to acquire these diseases.

You should restrict your consumption of sodium to fewer than 2300 mgs per day (that is about one teaspoon of salt) from all your foods. You should eat even less sodium if you've got high blood pressure, osteoporosis, kidney disease or diabetes.

The most effective method to control your sodium consumption is to consume fresh vegetables and fruits more frequently and prepare your own food. Try not to rely on frozen dinners or canned soup, meat or vegetables, as most bear a great deal of excess salt. If you do however purchase these foods, search for labels that read "no salt added" or "low sodium." Just look out for labels that read "reduced sodium" or "less salt," since the food might still have a high amount of salt.

Low Salt Tips

- Don't add salt while cooking

- While you're dining out, ask the cook to hold the salt.

- Remove the saltshaker off the dining table.

- Replace other seasonings for salt, like herbs, dry mustard, spices, lemon juice, ginger or garlic.

• Pick out fresh food as frequently as possible

• Avoid frozen dinners.

• Rinse off canned foods, like salmon, tuna fish and beans, under water to get rid of the salt.

• Avoid "instant" foods, including instant soups, oatmeal, pancakes and waffles.

• Avoid processed cheese.

• Avoid meats that have been processed, cured, or smoked.

• These include sausages, hot dogs, ham, bacon, pepperoni or smoked fish.

• Restrict snack foods, like salted crackers, chips, popcorn and salty nuts.

Chapter 7 – Valuable Tips to Losing Weight

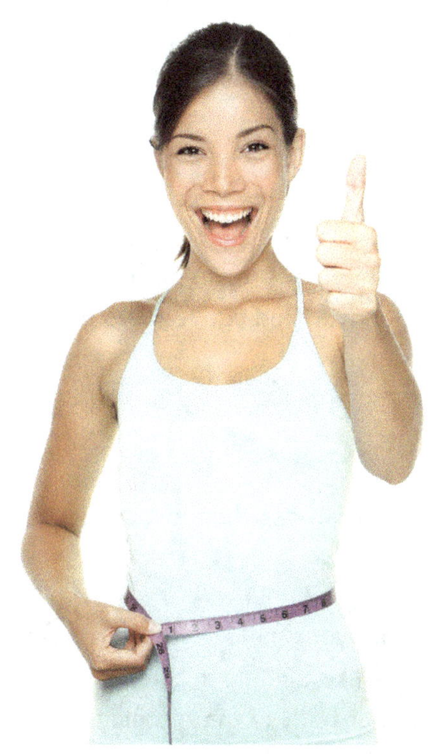

A fit weight is the key to a healthy maturing.

You may put on weight because:

- You eat too many calories. Perhaps you're dining out several times a week, consuming portions that are too big, snacking too frequently on high-fat foods or consuming drinks that hold a lot of sugar.

- You're not active enough and inactive people are more plausible to carry extra amounts body fat.

- You're losing muscle and acquiring fat as your metabolism decelerates.

Since muscle assists in burning calories, you'll discover that it is more difficult to burn off what you consume. At the same time, your body requires fewer calories the more you age, even if you're active.

The Secret is Variety

Whenever you consume an assortment of different foods, you will not feel bored or deprived and you're more plausible to acquire all the nutrients you require.

Don't Skip Breakfast

Consuming breakfast is among the most crucial things you are able to do to lose weight.

During the nighttime, your metabolism decelerates. Consuming a balanced breakfast - like high-fiber cereal, fruit and milk - assists you to jump-start your body in the morning and it will burn fuel a lot more effectively throughout the day.

Include High-Fiber Foods in Every Meal Plan

You'll find you are less hungry if you consume additional vegetables, fruit, legumes (like beans, lentils and chickpeas), as well as whole grains. Always consume three meals and two to three snacks daily. Once you have skipped a meal or snack, you will often consume more at the next one too frequently.

Monitor Your Fats

Since you require some fat to remain healthy, make certain you select healthy fats rather than unhealthy fats. Unhealthy fats are saturated and Trans fats. Healthy fats include monounsaturated and polyunsaturated fats. They could really cut down your cholesterol levels and your chance for heart disease and stroke. Healthy fats are found in vegetable oils, fish, nuts and seeds; even so, since nuts and seeds are as well high in calories, consume them in low amounts.

Aim for Only a Couple Calories in a Day

To sustain your weight, you want to burn off the same amount of calories you consume. Merely a couple of additional calories daily can tip the balance. If you add the daily excess of one hundred calories daily, then you'll end up with a sum of up to ten pounds of additional weight by the end of a year. That is a piece of bread and margarine, one scoop of ice cream or one can of soda per day.

But if you are able to scratch out those additional calories, or do more to burn them up, there is no reason you cannot keep up your weight or even drop off a couple of pounds. Clean out your cupboards and make the healthy selection the simple selection.

Control your Portions

Just about all people underrate the amount of food they consume daily by as much as one-third. For instance, a portion of fresh veggies amounts to a half a cup of broccoli, one portion of grains amounts to a half a cup of brown rice or pasta, one portion of meat is two-and-a-half ounces of lean beef and so forth.

Choose Your Fluids

What you drink may be just as significant as what you consume. Only one soft drink daily can accumulate to ten pounds yearly.

Regular soft drinks, fruit juice and alcohol are all high in calories (soft drinks, particularly, can also add to tooth disintegration).

Even coffee and tea may be packed with calories if you add sugar, cream or whole milk. As well, fancy coffees, liked flavored lattes and cappuccinos, can be as calorie-rich as a piece of cake.

ABOUT THE AUTHOR

Father-of-one Billy Joseph is a nutritionist. He creates recipes designed for weight loss. His clients include celebrities, politicians and the rich families of Miami, Florida.

Billy grew up in a vegan home, with both parents following the diet. He was introduced to vegan diet early but soon realized that there are other ways to still indulge the palates but regretting the decision to eat afterwards. That is when he decided to create delicious meals that don't only taste good but feel good too.

www.ingramcontent.com/pod-product-compliance
Lightning Source LLC
Chambersburg PA
CBHW050706250726
48662CB00002B/874